Summary

1.

2.

3.

4.

      a.

      b.

      c.

      d.

      e.

      f.

      g.

      h.

      i.

      j.

      k.

      l.

      m.

      n.

      o.

      p.

      q.

      r.

      s.

"Small Changes, Big Results: The Power of Habits"

Marc Ferrari

"Habit allows us to go from 'before' to 'after,' to make life easier and better.
Habit is notorious - and rightly so - for its ability to direct our actions,
even against our will; but by mindfully shaping our habits, we can harness the power of mindlessness as a sweeping force for serenity, energy, and growth."

Gretchen Rubin - Author, Podcaster and Speaker

Small Changes, Big Results: The Power of Habits

The Power of Habits:
How Small Changes Can Have Big Results

Hey there! We all have habits, whether we realize it or not. Habits are those things we do automatically, without much thought or effort. They can be good or bad, but one thing is for sure: they have a huge impact on our daily lives. That's why understanding the power of habits is so important if you want to make positive changes in your life.

Did you know that up to 45% of our daily behaviors are habitual? That's right, almost half of the things we do each day are on autopilot. That's why habits are so powerful - they shape our lives in ways we may not even realize. Think about it - if you have a habit of hitting the snooze button every morning, that can set the tone for a groggy, unproductive day. But if you have a habit of waking up early and going for a run, that can lead to increased energy, better focus, and improved mood.

The good news is that habits can be changed, and even small changes can have big results. This is because habits have a domino effect - one positive change can lead to other positive changes over time. For example, if you start with the small habit of drinking a glass of water every morning, that can lead to more energy, better digestion, and even weight loss. And once you see the positive effects of that one habit, you may be motivated to build on that success and create more positive habits in your life.

The key to harnessing the power of habits is to focus on the behaviors that will have the biggest impact on your life. This may mean identifying the habits that are holding you back, such as smoking or procrastination, and replacing them with new, positive habits. Or it may mean focusing on habits that will help you achieve your goals, such as setting a regular workout schedule or practicing a new skill every day.

When it comes to making changes to your habits, it's important to start small. Trying to overhaul your entire life at once is overwhelming and often leads to failure. Instead, focus on one small change at a time and build from there. This could mean something as simple as going to bed 10 minutes earlier each night or taking a short walk after dinner. Over time, these small changes will add up and create a positive ripple effect in your life.

Remember, the power of habits lies in their ability to shape our daily lives. By understanding the impact of habits and focusing on small changes, you can make a big impact on your life. So don't be afraid to start small and build from there. Every positive habit you create will have a cumulative effect on your overall well-being, leading to a happier, healthier, and more fulfilling life.

The Habit Loop:
Understanding the Science of Habit Formation

In order to understand how to build good habits, it's important to dive deeper into the science of habit formation. Habits are the small, automatic behaviors that we engage in on a daily basis - things like brushing our teeth, checking our phones, or snacking on junk food. These habits are created by the habit loop, which is a three-step process that begins with a cue, leads to a routine, and ends with a reward.

The first part of the habit loop is the cue. The cue is a trigger that signals to our brain that it's time to start the habit. Cues can be anything from a time of day, to a certain location, to an emotional state. For example, your cue to check your phone might be the sound of a notification, or your cue to eat junk food might be a stressful day at work.

Next up is the routine. The routine is the behavior itself - the habit that you want to change or establish. This is the action that you take in response to the cue. For example, if your cue is a stressful day at work, your routine might be to eat a bag of chips to help you feel better.

Finally, there's the reward. The reward is the positive outcome that you receive from the behavior. This is what reinforces the habit and makes it more likely to be repeated in the future. For example, the reward for eating the bag of chips might be a temporary feeling of satisfaction or relief from stress.

To change a habit, you need to disrupt the habit loop. This means identifying the cue that triggers the behavior, and finding a new routine that will lead to the same reward. For example, if you want to break the habit of eating junk food, you could try replacing it with a healthier routine, like going for a walk or doing some deep breathing exercises. These new routines can still provide the same reward of feeling better, but in a healthier way.

It's important to remember that breaking old habits and establishing new ones takes time and effort. According to research, it takes an average of 66 days for a new behavior to become automatic. So be patient with yourself and don't get discouraged if you don't see results right away.

Another important aspect of the habit loop is the role of cravings. Cravings are the intense desires or urges that we feel when we want to engage in a particular behavior. They can be triggered by cues in the environment, such as the sight or smell of food. To overcome cravings, it's important to have a plan in place. This could mean avoiding certain triggers, distracting yourself with another activity, or simply waiting it out until the craving subsides.

By understanding the habit loop, you can start to identify the specific cues, routines, and rewards that make up your own habits. With this knowledge, you can begin to create new, healthier habits by finding new routines that lead to the same rewards. And by overcoming cravings and sticking with your new habits, you can create positive changes in your life that will last. So go ahead and put the habit loop to work for you, and start building those good habits today!

Why Habits Matter:
The Benefits of Positive Habits

Habits are an integral part of our daily lives. From the moment we wake up until the moment we go to bed, we engage in various habits, both consciously and unconsciously. These habits range from brushing our teeth in the morning to checking our phones before bed. While some of our habits may be unintentional, others can be developed intentionally to improve our overall well-being.

Positive habits can have a powerful impact on our physical health. Regular exercise, healthy eating habits, and getting enough sleep are just a few examples of positive habits that can help us maintain a healthy weight, reduce the risk of chronic diseases, and improve our overall energy levels. By making these habits a part of our daily routine, we can enjoy the many physical benefits that come with them.

In addition to physical health, positive habits can also have a profound impact on our mental and emotional well-being. Habits such as practicing gratitude, meditating, or journaling can help us reduce stress, improve our mood, and build greater resilience in the face of challenges. By taking care of our mental and emotional health through positive habits, we can improve our overall quality of life and be better equipped to handle the ups and downs of daily life.

Positive habits can also have a ripple effect on other areas of our lives. For example, developing the habit of regular exercise can lead to greater self-confidence and a sense of accomplishment, which can spill over into other areas of our lives. Similarly, the habit of practicing gratitude can lead to more positive relationships with others, as we become more appreciative and grateful for the people in our lives.

Another benefit of positive habits is that they can help us achieve our goals. By breaking down our goals into smaller, more manageable steps and turning those steps into habits, we can make progress towards our goals without feeling overwhelmed. For example, if your goal is to write a book, you might turn the habit of writing for 30 minutes every day into a regular part of your routine. By doing this, you can make steady progress towards your goal without feeling like you have to do everything at once.

Finally, positive habits can help us build a sense of purpose and meaning in our lives. By developing habits that align with our values and goals, we can create a sense of direction and purpose that can guide us through the ups and downs of daily life. Whether it's volunteering regularly, practicing a creative hobby, or learning something new, positive habits can help us feel more connected to ourselves and the world around us.

It's important to note that developing positive habits is not a one-size-fits-all solution. Different habits work for different people, and it's up to each individual to figure out which habits work best for them. It's also important to remember that developing positive habits takes time and effort. It's not something that happens overnight, but with consistent practice and patience, positive habits can become a natural part of our daily routine.

Positive habits matter because they can improve our physical health, mental and emotional well-being, relationships, goal achievement, and sense of purpose. By focusing on developing and maintaining positive habits, we can create positive changes in our lives that will last. So go ahead and start building those good habits today - your body, mind, and spirit will thank you for it!

Identifying Your Habits:
Self-Awareness for Habit Change

Habits are a part of our daily routine, often so ingrained that we don't even realize we're doing them. They can be positive, like exercising or meditating, or negative, like smoking or overeating. But whether positive or negative, our habits have a powerful impact on our lives, shaping our health, relationships, and overall well-being.

To change our habits, we first need to become more self-aware of the habits we currently engage in. By identifying our habits and understanding the underlying factors that contribute to them, we can start to make positive changes and create new, healthier habits.

The first step in identifying our habits is to observe ourselves. Pay attention to your daily routines and the things you do throughout the day. What are your go-to behaviors in response to different situations? When do you engage in certain behaviors? For example, do you reach for a cigarette when you feel stressed, or do you turn to social media when you're bored?

Keeping a habit journal or using a habit tracking app can be a helpful way to record your actions throughout the day and identify patterns in your behavior. You might be surprised at how much you do without even realizing it!

Once you've identified your habits, it's important to understand the triggers that lead to those habits. Habits are often formed in response to specific cues, such as stress, boredom, or hunger. By understanding what triggers our habits, we can start to develop strategies to change them. For example, if you tend to snack when you're feeling stressed, you can try to find other ways to cope with stress, such as taking a walk or practicing deep breathing exercises.

Another important aspect of self-awareness for habit change is understanding the rewards we receive from our habits. Habits are often formed because they provide some form of reward, whether it's a sense of satisfaction, relief from stress, or a quick energy boost. By understanding the rewards we receive from our habits, we can start to find alternative behaviors that provide similar rewards. For example, if you tend to reach for sugary snacks for a quick energy boost, you can try eating a piece of fruit or taking a quick walk instead.

Self-awareness is also important for identifying the beliefs and values that underpin our habits. Our habits are often tied to our beliefs about ourselves and the world around us. For example, if we believe that we're not good at public speaking, we may avoid opportunities to speak in public, which can become a habit over time. By identifying these underlying beliefs, we can start to challenge them and develop new, more positive beliefs that support the habits we want to develop.

Finally, self-awareness is important for developing self-compassion as we work to change our habits. Developing new habits takes time and effort, and it's important to be patient and kind to ourselves throughout the process. By being self-aware of our habits and the challenges we face in changing them, we can practice self-compassion and avoid self-criticism.

Self-awareness is a key component of habit change. By identifying our habits, understanding their triggers and rewards, and being aware of the beliefs and values that underpin them, we can start to make positive changes in our lives. With patience, self-compassion, and a commitment to self-awareness, we can develop the habits that support our overall well-being and happiness.

Habit Stacking:
Building Positive Habits One Step at a Time

If you've ever tried to make a big change in your life, you know how challenging it can be. Whether you're trying to lose weight, quit smoking, or start a new exercise routine, it can be difficult to stick to new habits consistently. That's where the concept of habit stacking comes in. Habit stacking is a simple and effective way to build positive habits one step at a time.

The basic idea behind habit stacking is to use an existing habit as a trigger for a new habit. When we anchor a new habit to an existing habit, it becomes easier to remember and more likely to stick. The key is to choose a simple and consistent trigger, something we do every day without fail.

For example, let's say you want to start a new habit of doing a daily meditation practice. You might choose to anchor this new habit to an existing habit, such as brushing your teeth in the morning. You could decide to meditate for just one minute after you finish brushing your teeth. Over time, as you become accustomed to the new habit, you can gradually increase the duration of your meditation practice.

Habit stacking works because it leverages the power of our existing habits. By building on habits that we're already doing consistently, we're less likely to forget or skip the new habit. We also reduce the cognitive load of trying to remember a new behavior and create a new routine.

Instead, the new habit becomes a natural part of our existing routine.

To use habit stacking effectively, it's important to choose the right trigger and make the new habit as simple and easy as possible. The new habit should be something that can be completed quickly and easily, without requiring a lot of time or effort. For example, if you want to develop the habit of reading every day, you could anchor it to your lunch break or your commute to work. You could decide to read just one page or one chapter each day, making it easy to fit into your routine.

Habit stacking can also be used to build a chain of positive habits. Once you've established one habit, you can use it as a trigger for the next habit. For example, if you've established a habit of doing a daily meditation practice, you could use that habit as a trigger for a new habit of doing a few stretches or exercises. Over time, you can continue to add new habits to your routine, building a chain of positive habits that support your overall well-being and happiness.

By building positive habits one step at a time, you can make sustainable changes in your life without feeling overwhelmed or discouraged. With habit stacking, you can break down big goals into smaller, more manageable steps, creating a sense of progress and momentum. This can be especially helpful when you're trying to establish new habits that may not come naturally to you.

It's important to note that habit stacking is not a magic bullet that will make habit change effortless. Like any change, it requires effort and commitment. But by leveraging the power of our existing habits and making the new habits as simple and easy as possible, we can set ourselves up for success.

Habit stacking is a powerful tool for building positive habits one step at a time. By anchoring a new habit to an existing habit, we make it easier to remember and more likely to stick. By choosing simple and easy habits, we reduce the cognitive load of creating a new routine. By building a chain of positive habits, we create a foundation of well-being and happiness in our lives. With habit stacking, we can achieve our goals and create the life we want, one small step at a time.

Breaking Bad Habits:
Strategies for Overcoming Negative Behaviors

Breaking a bad habit can be a difficult process, but it's one that is definitely worth the effort. Whether it's biting your nails, procrastinating, or indulging in unhealthy foods, bad habits can have a negative impact on our health, relationships, and overall well-being. Fortunately, there are many strategies you can use to break a bad habit and establish new, healthier behaviors.

The first step in breaking a bad habit is to identify the triggers that cause the behavior. These triggers can be internal, such as stress or boredom, or external, such as social situations or the availability of the habit-forming substance. Once you have identified your triggers, you can develop strategies to avoid or manage them. For example, if you tend to snack on junk food when you're stressed, you might try exercising or meditating instead.

Simply trying to stop a bad habit may not be enough. It's important to replace the habit with a healthier alternative. For example, if you're trying to quit smoking, you might replace the habit with exercise or deep breathing exercises to manage cravings. If you're trying to stop snacking on unhealthy foods, you might replace the habit with healthy snacks, such as fruits or vegetables.

Using positive self-talk is another powerful strategy for breaking a bad habit. Our thoughts and beliefs can influence our behavior, so it's important to reinforce the idea that you can succeed. Rather than telling yourself that you can't break the habit, tell yourself that you are capable of change and that you are making progress. Enlisting the support of friends, family, or a therapist is also a great way to stay motivated and accountable.

Visualization is another powerful tool for breaking a bad habit. By visualizing yourself successfully breaking the habit, you can rewire your brain and make the new habit feel more natural. Imagine yourself in situations that would normally trigger the behavior, but this time, imagine yourself choosing a healthier alternative.

It's also important to make small, gradual changes to your behavior. Trying to make too many changes at once can be overwhelming and set you up for failure. For example, if you're trying to cut back on your alcohol consumption, you might start by having one less drink each week until you reach your goal.

Finally, it's important to be patient and persistent when breaking a bad habit. It's not an overnight process, and there may be setbacks and slip-ups along the way. But don't be discouraged - use these as opportunities to learn and grow. Focus on the benefits of breaking the habit, such as improved health, more time, and better relationships, and keep your eye on the end goal.

Breaking a bad habit is a challenging process, but it's one that is definitely worth the effort. By identifying triggers, replacing the habit with a healthier alternative, using positive self-talk, enlisting support, using visualization techniques, making small changes, and being patient and persistent, you can overcome negative behaviors and establish new, healthier habits. Remember that the journey to breaking a bad habit is just as important as the end result. With the right strategies and mindset, you can achieve your goal and create positive changes in your life.

Creating Habits That Stick:
Tips for Long-Term Success

Creating habits that stick can be challenging, but it's an important part of achieving lasting change. Many people start off strong when trying to establish new habits, but struggle to maintain them over time. However, by following a few key strategies, you can increase your chances of success and build habits that stick.

One of the most important factors in creating habits that stick is consistency. This means performing your new habit regularly, ideally on a daily basis. Consistency helps to create new neural pathways in the brain, making the habit easier to perform over time. It's important to remember that forming a new habit takes time and effort, but with consistency, it will eventually become easier and more automatic.

Setting realistic goals is also essential to creating habits that stick. Starting small and gradually increasing the difficulty of the habit can help to ensure success and avoid overwhelming yourself. Setting achievable goals will build your confidence and make it easier to maintain the habit in the long term.

Accountability can also be a powerful tool in creating habits that stick. Having someone to hold you accountable can help to keep you motivated and committed to your new habit. This might mean finding a friend or family member who can check in on your progress, joining an accountability group or working with a coach.

Creating a supportive environment can also be key to building habits that stick. This means surrounding yourself with people who support and encourage your new habit, and removing any barriers or distractions that might get in the way of your progress. For example, if you're trying to establish a new exercise routine, finding a workout buddy or joining a fitness class can provide the social support you need to stay on track.

Celebrating your progress and rewarding yourself for your efforts is another important strategy for creating habits that stick. Small rewards, such as treating yourself to a movie or your favorite food, can help to build momentum and motivation for sticking with the habit. Celebrating your progress can also help to reinforce the habit and make it more enjoyable.

Finally, it's important to have a plan for when setbacks occur. Anticipating obstacles and having a strategy in place for how to handle them can help to prevent setbacks from derailing your progress. This might mean adjusting your expectations, seeking additional support or finding alternative ways to perform the habit.

Creating habits that stick requires consistency, setting realistic goals, creating accountability, building a supportive environment, celebrating progress and having a plan for setbacks. By following these strategies, you can build habits that become a natural part of your daily routine and achieve your goals. Remember that forming a new habit takes time and effort, but with patience and persistence, you can create lasting change.

The Role of Willpower in Habit Formation: How to Strengthen Your Resolve

Willpower is a complex and essential element of habit formation. It's the inner strength that allows you to push through distractions, overcome temptation, and stay focused on your goals. Willpower is also a limited resource, which means that if you're not careful, it can be depleted quickly. However, with the right strategies and habits, you can strengthen your willpower and make it work for you, rather than against you.

One key way to strengthen your willpower is to set clear and specific goals. When you have a specific target in mind, it becomes much easier to stay motivated and focused on the task at hand. For example, if your goal is to start a regular exercise habit, you might set a specific goal to exercise for 30 minutes every morning.

Another way to build willpower is through self-care. This means taking care of yourself physically and emotionally by getting enough sleep, eating a healthy diet, and managing stress. When you take care of yourself, you're better equipped to deal with the challenges that come with habit formation.

Creating a supportive environment is also crucial for building willpower. This might mean finding a friend or family member who supports your goals, joining a community of like-minded individuals, or seeking out a coach or mentor who can provide guidance and support.

Practicing mindfulness is another powerful way to strengthen your willpower. Mindfulness is the practice of being present in the moment, without judgment. When you practice mindfulness, you become more aware of your thoughts and feelings, and you can choose to respond to them in a more intentional way. This can help you to resist temptation and stay focused on your goals.

In addition to these strategies, there are other steps you can take to build your willpower. For example, taking breaks when you need them, avoiding decision fatigue, and breaking down large goals into smaller, more manageable ones can all help you stay on track.

It's important to be kind and compassionate to yourself as you work on building your willpower. Habits take time to form, and setbacks and challenges are a normal part of the process. By celebrating your successes, even the small ones, and being patient and persistent in your efforts, you can build the willpower you need to achieve your goals and create the life you desire.

Building willpower is essential for forming and maintaining positive habits. By setting clear goals, practicing self-care, creating a supportive environment, practicing mindfulness, and being patient and persistent in your efforts, you can strengthen your willpower and increase your chances of success. Remember that building willpower takes time, effort, and dedication, but with the right approach, you can achieve anything you set your mind   to.

Tracking Your Habits:
Tools and Techniques for Monitoring Progress

Tracking your habits is a valuable technique for forming positive habits and achieving your goals. It helps you stay focused and motivated by providing a clear overview of your progress, and it can also help you identify areas for improvement. In this chapter, we'll explore some effective tools and techniques for tracking your habits and monitoring your progress in greater detail.

One popular and simple method for tracking your habits is to use a habit tracker. This tool allows you to record your progress each day for the habits you're working on. Habit tracker apps and templates are available online, or you can create your own using a notebook or planner. The key is to find a system that works for you and use it consistently.

When using a habit tracker, it's important to be specific and realistic about the habits you're tracking. Instead of tracking broad habits like "exercise," break them down into more specific actions like "30 minutes of cardio," or "10,000 steps." This helps you see your progress and identify areas for improvement more clearly.

A habit journal is another effective tool for tracking your habits. It's a more detailed approach that lets you reflect on your progress, patterns, and triggers affecting your habits. In your habit journal, you might record how you feel each day, any obstacles you faced, and the strategies you used to overcome them. This kind of reflection allows you to spot trends, understand what's working for you, and adjust your habits accordingly.

Visual cues can also be used to track your habits, such as sticky notes or whiteboards. These reminders can help keep your habits in focus and provide an additional level of accountability. For habits that require daily repetition, like flossing or meditation, having a visual cue can be especially effective.

It's important to avoid becoming overly focused on the data when tracking your habits. While tracking your progress is important, it's also important to stay focused on your overall goals and celebrate your successes along the way. Don't get discouraged by occasional setbacks or fluctuations in your progress. Remember that habit formation is a process, and it's important to enjoy the journey.

One final consideration when tracking your habits is to stay flexible and adaptable. If a particular habit tracker or tool isn't working for you, don't hesitate to try something new. The most important thing is to find a system that works for you and stick with it consistently over time.

Tracking your habits is a valuable tool for successful habit formation. By using a habit tracker, habit journal, or other tracking tool, you can monitor your progress, identify areas for improvement, and stay motivated as you work towards your goals. Remember to be specific and realistic about your habits, celebrate your successes, and stay flexible and adaptable as you navigate the habit formation process. With these tools and techniques, you'll be well on your way to creating the habits you need to achieve your dreams and live the life you desire.

The Social Side of Habits:
Building Habits with Support and
Accountability

As humans, we are social creatures, and building habits with the support of others can make all the difference in our success. Not only does having a support system provide accountability, but it can also be a source of motivation and inspiration. Research has shown that people who have support and accountability when trying to make a change are more likely to stick to their goals and see lasting results.

When building habits with support, it's essential to find people who share your values and goals. This can be a friend, family member, coworker, or someone you meet through a group or online community. Look for people who are positive, supportive, and committed to making positive changes in their own lives.

Communicating your goals clearly is also key when building habits with support. Be honest about what you're trying to achieve and what kind of support you need. Let your support system know how often you'd like to check in, what kind of feedback you're looking for, and what kind of support you need when you're struggling.

To create a supportive community, consider starting a group or joining one that already exists. This can be an online community, a local group, or a group of friends who are committed to supporting each other in achieving their goals. Social media can also be a great tool for finding like-minded people who are working on similar habits.

It's important to remember that building habits with support isn't just about receiving help, but also about providing it. Be a positive and encouraging influence on others in your support system. Celebrate their successes, provide feedback, and offer words of encouragement when they're struggling. Remember that when you support others, you're also building a community that will be there for you when you need it.

If you're struggling to find a support system or need additional guidance, consider working with a coach or therapist who specializes in habit formation. These professionals can provide expert guidance, support, and accountability to help you achieve your goals.

Building habits with support and accountability can be a powerful tool for habit formation. When you have a community of positive and supportive people, you're more likely to stick to your habits and make meaningful changes. Be clear about your goals and what kind of support you need, and be a positive influence on others in your support system. With the right support, you can build the habits you need to achieve your dreams and live the life   you   desire.

The Keystone Habit: How One Small Change Can Transform Your Life

Have you ever wondered why it's so hard to make lasting changes in your life? You start off with good intentions, but before you know it, you've fallen back into your old habits. The key to making lasting changes is to identify your keystone habit - that one small change that can have a big impact on your life.

The concept of the keystone habit was popularized by author Charles Duhigg in his book "The Power of Habit." Duhigg defines a keystone habit as a "small win" that creates a positive ripple effect in other areas of your life. Keystone habits are like the foundation of a house - if they're solid, everything else will fall into place.

To find your keystone habit, think about the changes you want to make in your life and the areas you want to improve. Then, identify the habits that could have a positive ripple effect on those areas. For example, if you want to improve your physical health, your keystone habit could be to exercise every morning. If you want to improve your mental health, your keystone habit could be to meditate for 10 minutes every day.

The key to making your keystone habit stick is to start small and be consistent. Instead of trying to make too many changes at once, focus on building one new habit at a time. Choose a small change that you can easily incorporate into your daily routine, and commit to practicing it every day for at least 30 days. Research has shown that it takes an average of 66 days to form a new habit, so be patient and persistent.

Another way to make your keystone habit stick is to create a trigger for it. A trigger is a cue that reminds you to do your habit. For example, if your keystone habit is to exercise every morning, you could set your workout clothes out the night before or place your sneakers by your bed to remind you to exercise.

In addition to creating triggers, it's important to track your progress. Use a habit tracker app or a simple notebook to record your daily progress. Seeing your progress over time can be incredibly motivating and can help you stay committed to your keystone habit.

Remember, your keystone habit is just the beginning. As you continue to practice your habit, you'll start to see positive changes in other areas of your life. Your keystone habit can be the catalyst for a positive feedback loop that leads to lasting change and a happier, healthier you. So start small, be consistent, and watch as your keystone habit transforms your life.

Mindful Habits:
The Benefits of Bringing Awareness to Your Behaviors

Introduction:

In our busy lives, it's easy to slip into autopilot mode and let our habits control our actions without much thought. However, developing mindfulness in our habits can help us lead a more intentional and fulfilling life. In this chapter, we will discuss the benefits of mindful habits and explore ways to incorporate mindfulness into our daily routines.

The Importance of Mindfulness:

Mindfulness is the practice of being present and fully engaged in the current moment. When we apply this practice to our habits, we become more aware of our actions and the impact they have on our lives. By paying attention to our habits, we can identify which ones are serving us and which ones are holding us back.

For example, if we mindlessly snack throughout the day, we may not realize how many calories we are consuming. However, if we bring mindfulness to our eating habits, we can savor the taste of each bite and better tune in to our hunger and fullness signals. This can lead to more balanced and healthy eating habits.

Benefits of Mindful Habits:

- Improved Self-Awareness: Mindful habits require us to pay attention to our thoughts, emotions, and actions. This increased self-awareness can help us identify patterns in our behaviors and make positive changes.

- Reduced Stress: Mindfulness has been shown to reduce stress and anxiety levels. When we approach our habits with mindfulness, we are less likely to feel overwhelmed or rushed.

- Enhanced Focus: Mindfulness can improve our ability to focus and concentrate. By bringing our attention to our habits, we can eliminate distractions and fully engage in the task at hand.

- Increased Creativity: Mindfulness has been shown to enhance creativity and problem-solving abilities. By approaching our habits with curiosity and openness, we may discover new and innovative ways to approach our daily routines.

Incorporating Mindfulness into Your Habits:

- Start Small: Begin by bringing mindfulness to one habit at a time. This could be as simple as brushing your teeth or making your bed. Over time, you can gradually incorporate mindfulness into more areas of your life.

- Use Your Senses: Engage your senses to bring more awareness to your habits. For example, when eating, take the time to savor the flavors and textures of your food.

- Take Breaks: Build in breaks throughout the day to pause and check in with yourself. This can help you stay focused and reduce stress.

- Practice Gratitude: When we approach our habits with gratitude, we are more likely to approach them with a positive mindset. Take a moment to reflect on the benefits of the habit you are practicing.

Incorporating mindfulness into our habits can help us lead a more intentional and fulfilling life. By being present and fully engaged in the current moment, we can improve our self-awareness, reduce stress, enhance focus, and increase creativity. By starting small and using our senses, we can gradually incorporate mindfulness into our daily routines and reap the benefits of a more mindful and intentional life.

The Power of Habit Cues: How to Use Triggers for Positive Change

Habits are formed through a repetitive cycle of cue, routine, and reward. Understanding how this habit loop works can help you create new, positive habits in your life. A cue is a trigger or a reminder that initiates a behavior or routine. It can be anything from a sound, a smell, a time of day, a location, or even an emotion. Cues are the first step in creating a habit and play a critical role in habit formation.

When trying to create new habits, it is essential to identify and use the right cues that trigger the desired behavior. By using a specific cue, you can train your brain to automatically initiate the desired behavior or routine. For example, if you want to develop a habit of reading every night before bed, you can set a cue that triggers the behavior, such as placing the book on your bedside table or setting a reminder on your phone.

One effective way to use cues to build new habits is to piggyback on existing habits. For example, if you want to develop a habit of drinking more water, you can associate drinking water with an existing habit, such as brushing your teeth. After brushing your teeth, you can place a glass of water on your bathroom counter and drink it. By doing this consistently, you will create a new habit of drinking water after brushing your teeth.

It is essential to remember that cues can also trigger negative habits. For example, if you tend to snack on junk food when you are stressed, the feeling of stress can be the cue that triggers the habit. Identifying the cues that trigger negative habits is the first step in breaking the cycle.

Once you have identified the cue that triggers the habit, you can begin to replace the routine or behavior with a positive one. For example, if you tend to snack on junk food when you are stressed, you can replace the habit with a healthier alternative, such as going for a walk or doing some deep breathing exercises.

It is also important to note that habits are not all or nothing. It is okay to slip up or miss a day, but it is crucial to get back on track and continue to practice the behavior consistently. By doing so, you strengthen the habit and make it more automatic.

Using the right cues is crucial to building positive habits. By identifying the cues that trigger the desired behavior, you can train your brain to initiate the behavior automatically. Piggybacking on existing habits and replacing negative behaviors with positive ones can help you achieve long-term success in habit formation. Remember that habits take time to form, so be patient and consistent, and eventually, your positive habits will become   second   nature.

Habits and Health:
The Connection Between Lifestyle Behaviors and Well-Being

Introduction:

The habits we form play a significant role in our overall health and well-being. Our daily routines and lifestyle behaviors have a direct impact on our physical, mental, and emotional health. From what we eat to how much we sleep, our habits can either promote or hinder our health. In this chapter, we will explore the connection between habits and health, and the importance of developing positive lifestyle behaviors to support optimal well-being.

The Impact of Habits on Health:

Our habits can affect many aspects of our health, including our weight, cardiovascular health, mental health, and overall longevity. Eating a healthy diet and engaging in regular physical activity can promote healthy weight and reduce the risk of chronic diseases such as diabetes, heart disease, and certain types of cancer. Similarly, getting enough sleep, managing stress, and engaging in positive social interactions can promote mental and emotional health, reducing the risk of depression, anxiety, and other mental health disorders.

The Importance of Positive Lifestyle Behaviors:

Developing positive lifestyle behaviors is key to promoting optimal health and well-being. Positive habits such as regular exercise, a healthy diet, getting enough sleep, and managing stress can help prevent disease, improve mental and emotional health, and increase overall longevity. Additionally, engaging in positive social interactions and finding ways to give back to the community can help promote a sense of purpose and meaning in life, which can further enhance overall well-being.

Tips for Developing Positive Habits for Health:

Developing positive habits for health can be challenging, especially when we are trying to break old, negative habits. Here are some tips for developing and maintaining positive lifestyle behaviors:

- Start small: Choose one habit to focus on at a time, and start with a small change. For example, try replacing one unhealthy snack with a healthy option, or going for a short walk each day.

- Be consistent: Consistency is key when it comes to developing habits. Try to stick to your new habit for at least 21 days to give it a chance to become a part of your routine.

- Find support: Enlist the help of friends or family members to help keep you accountable and motivated in developing positive habits.

- Be patient: Developing new habits takes time, so be patient with yourself and celebrate small victories along the way.

Our daily habits and lifestyle behaviors have a significant impact on our overall health and well-being. Developing positive habits for health, such as regular exercise, a healthy diet, getting enough sleep, and managing stress, can help promote optimal health and reduce the risk of chronic diseases. By making small changes and being consistent, we can develop positive habits that support our well-being and lead to a more fulfilling life.

Financial Habits:
How Money Habits Impact Your Financial Health

Introduction:

Your financial health is just as important as your physical and mental health. The way you manage your money can have a significant impact on your overall well-being. Good financial habits can help you stay on top of your finances, avoid debt, and achieve your financial goals. In this chapter, we will explore the importance of financial habits, how they can impact your financial health, and some practical tips for developing and maintaining healthy financial habits.

The Importance of Financial Habits:

Your financial habits are the small decisions you make every day that impact your financial situation. These habits can be as simple as making a cup of coffee at home instead of buying one on the way to work or as significant as putting a portion of your paycheck into a savings account each month. Developing and maintaining healthy financial habits is essential because they can help you:

- Stay on top of your finances
- Avoid debt and financial stress
- Build wealth and achieve your financial goals
- Maintain a good credit score
- Be prepared for unexpected expenses or emergencies

How Financial Habits Impact Your Financial Health:

Your financial habits can impact your financial health in several ways. For example, if you consistently overspend or fail to save, you may find yourself in debt or struggling to pay bills. On the other hand, if you make a habit of saving and investing, you can build wealth over time and achieve your financial goals. Additionally, your financial habits can impact your credit score, which can impact your ability to get loans or credit cards at a reasonable rate.

Developing Healthy Financial Habits:

Developing healthy financial habits takes time and effort, but it is worth it in the long run. Here are some practical tips for developing and maintaining healthy financial habits:

- Create a Budget: Creating a budget is an essential step in developing healthy financial habits. Start by listing your income and expenses, then allocate your income to cover your expenses while leaving some money for saving and investing.

- Track Your Spending: Tracking your spending can help you identify areas where you may be overspending or where you can make cutbacks. There are several apps and tools available that can help you track your spending and manage your finances.

- Automate Your Savings: Automating your savings can make it easier to save money regularly. Set up automatic transfers to your savings account each month to make saving a habit.

- Pay Yourself First: Make a habit of paying yourself first by setting aside a portion of your income for savings and investing before paying bills or other expenses.

- Pay Your Debt: Making a habit of limiting your debt can help you avoid financial stress and keep your credit score in good standing. Make sure to pay your bills on time, avoid high-interest loans, and limit your use of credit cards. Start planning to pay in full for everything you buy and make a plan to pay your debts. You may start paying from the smallest to largest, and each debt you pay will be a small win to you towards a Debt Free position.

Developing healthy financial habits is essential for your financial well-being. Your financial habits impact your financial health, so it's important to make positive financial habits a priority. By creating a budget, tracking your spending, automating your savings, paying yourself first, and limiting your debt, you can develop and maintain healthy financial habits that will benefit you in the long run. Remember, good financial habits take time and effort to develop, but the results are worth it.

The Impact of Digital Habits:
How to Build a Healthy Relationship with Technology

In today's world, it's hard to imagine life without technology. From smartphones and laptops to social media and video streaming, we rely on digital tools and platforms to stay connected, informed, and entertained. While technology has many benefits, it's important to be mindful of how our digital habits impact our well-being. In this chapter, we'll explore the impact of digital habits and provide tips for building a healthy relationship with technology.

The Pros and Cons of Digital Habits

There's no denying that technology has changed our lives in many positive ways. It has made it easier to stay in touch with loved ones, access information, and complete tasks more efficiently. However, there are also downsides to our reliance on technology. For example, excessive screen time has been linked to poor sleep quality, eye strain, and mental health issues such as anxiety and depression. It's important to be aware of the potential negative effects of digital habits and take steps to mitigate them.

Building Healthy Digital Habits

The good news is that it's possible to build healthy digital habits that promote well-being. Here are some tips for doing so:

- Set Boundaries: Set clear boundaries for your digital use. For example, you might decide to avoid checking your phone during meals or before bedtime. It's also helpful to turn off notifications for non-essential apps and limit your overall screen time.

- Practice Mindful Consumption: Be mindful of what you're consuming online. Avoid mindlessly scrolling through social media feeds and instead, make a conscious effort to engage with content that adds value to your life.

- Take Breaks: Take regular breaks from technology throughout the day. This might mean going for a walk, reading a book, or spending time with loved ones. It's important to give your brain a break from the constant stimulation of digital devices.

- Use Technology to Support Your Goals: Instead of mindlessly consuming content, use technology to support your goals. For example, you might use a fitness app to track your workouts or a productivity app to manage your to-do list.

- Seek Support: If you find it difficult to build healthy digital habits on your own, seek support from others. Join a support group, talk to a therapist, or enlist the help of a friend or family member to hold you accountable.

In today's digital age, it's important to be mindful of our technology use and its impact on our well-being. By setting boundaries, practicing mindful consumption, taking breaks, using technology to support our goals, and seeking support, we can build healthy digital habits that promote overall health and happiness. So, let's make a conscious effort to build a healthy relationship with technology and use it as a tool for growth and fulfillment, rather than a source of stress and distraction.

Habits and Relationships: Building Positive Habits for Stronger Connections

Relationships are a fundamental part of our lives, and the habits we form can have a profound impact on our interactions with others. Building positive habits can help us create stronger connections and deepen our relationships with loved ones, friends, and colleagues.

The first step in building positive relationship habits is to understand the importance of consistency. Consistency is key to building and maintaining any habit, and it's especially important in relationships. Small, consistent actions can help us develop a sense of trust and reliability with the people in our lives. For example, consistently following through on commitments, showing up on time, and being present during conversations can help us build stronger connections.

Another important aspect of building positive relationship habits is understanding the power of positivity. When we focus on positive interactions with others, we can create a virtuous cycle of positivity that can lead to stronger relationships. Simple acts of kindness, like expressing gratitude or offering words of encouragement, can go a long way in building positive relationships. It's important to remember that these small acts don't need to be grand gestures, but rather consistent actions that show we care.

One key habit that can improve relationships is active listening. Active listening means being fully present and engaged in the conversation, seeking to understand the other person's perspective, and validating their feelings. When we actively listen, we can build stronger connections and create a sense of trust and understanding. In contrast, when we fail to listen, we may miss important cues and misunderstand the needs and feelings of others.

It's also important to identify any negative relationship habits we may have and work to change them. Negative habits, such as always interrupting others or being consistently late, can damage relationships and erode trust. Identifying and changing these negative habits can help us create stronger and healthier connections with those around us.

Finally, it's important to recognize that building positive relationship habits takes time and effort. It requires a commitment to consistently practicing positive actions and behaviors, even when it's difficult or uncomfortable. But the rewards of building positive relationship habits are well worth the effort, as they can help us create deeper connections with those around us and enrich our lives in countless ways.

Building positive relationship habits is essential for creating stronger connections with the people in our lives. By focusing on consistency, positivity, active listening, and identifying and changing negative habits, we can build stronger and healthier relationships. Remember, building positive relationship habits takes time and effort, but the rewards are immeasurable.

Building Habits for Work and Productivity: Strategies for Getting Things Done

Habits play an essential role in our personal and professional lives, including our work and productivity. Whether you are an entrepreneur, a freelancer, or an employee, cultivating positive habits can help you stay on track, increase your focus, and enhance your efficiency.

In this chapter, we'll explore some strategies for building habits that can help you achieve your goals and increase your productivity at work.

- Define your goals: Start by setting clear and specific goals that you want to achieve in your work. These goals should be measurable, achievable, and realistic. Once you have identified your goals, break them down into smaller tasks that you can work on each day.

- Create a routine: Develop a daily routine that is consistent and aligned with your goals. Determine the best time of day to work on each task, and stick to a schedule that works for you.

- Prioritize your tasks: Identify the most critical tasks that need to be completed first, and prioritize them accordingly. This will help you avoid procrastination and stay on track with your goals.

- Use technology to your advantage: Take advantage of productivity tools and software that can help you manage your tasks, track your progress, and stay organized. Some popular options include Trello, Asana, and Todoist.

- Break up big tasks: If a task seems overwhelming, break it down into smaller, more manageable tasks. This will help you stay focused and motivated, and ensure that you make progress towards your goals.

- Eliminate distractions: Identify any distractions that may be preventing you from being productive and eliminate them. This could include turning off your phone, blocking social media sites, or working in a quiet environment.

- Make it a habit: Consistency is key when it comes to building habits. Set aside time each day to work on your tasks, and make it a habit to stick to your routine. Over time, these positive habits will become ingrained, and you'll find that you are achieving your goals more easily and efficiently.

- Find an accountability partner: Having someone to hold you accountable can help you stay on track with your goals. Find a friend or colleague who is also interested in building productive habits and work together to stay motivated and on track.

Building positive habits can help you become more productive, efficient, and successful in your work. By setting clear goals, establishing a routine, prioritizing your tasks, using technology to your advantage, and eliminating distractions, you can build habits that will help you achieve your goals and lead to greater success. Remember, it takes time and consistency to build habits, but the results are well worth the effort.

Habit Formation for Creativity: How Habits Can Support Your Artistic Practice

In the world of art and creativity, it can be easy to get lost in the process and let go of structure. However, building positive habits can actually help support your artistic practice and enhance your creative output. In this chapter, we will explore the importance of habits in artistic work and how to develop effective habits for a more productive and fulfilling creative life.

The Importance of Habits in Artistic Practice

As an artist or creative, it can be tempting to think that structure and routine may stifle your creativity. However, habits can actually be a valuable tool in helping to enhance your creative output. By building habits, you can create a foundation of consistency and structure that supports your artistic process.

Habits can also help to eliminate the distractions and decisions that can prevent you from getting started on your creative work. When you establish a habit of working on your art at a certain time each day or week, it becomes easier to sit down and get started without the need to make decisions about when or where to work. This allows you to focus more on the creative process and less on logistical or administrative details.

Developing Effective Habits for Creativity

When it comes to building habits that support creativity, it's important to identify the specific areas where you want to establish consistency in your creative work. Here are some key steps to follow:

- Identify your creative goals: To start building effective habits, it's important to know what you want to achieve creatively. Set specific, measurable goals that are aligned with your long-term artistic vision.

- Determine your creative habits: Look for the actions that will help you achieve your goals. These could include working on your art at the same time each day, setting specific creative tasks for each session, or establishing a daily journaling practice to stimulate creativity.

- Start small: Begin by establishing one or two simple habits that you can realistically achieve. As you begin to establish these habits, gradually increase the complexity and frequency of your creative tasks.

- Use cues and rewards: Incorporate cues and rewards to help reinforce your habits. This could be as simple as setting a timer for your creative work, or rewarding yourself with a treat or activity once you complete a certain number of creative tasks.

- Stay accountable: Share your goals and progress with others, whether through an artistic community or with friends and family. This can help you stay accountable to your creative goals and motivate you to continue building effective habits.

Building effective habits can be a powerful tool in supporting your artistic practice and enhancing your creativity. By establishing consistency and structure in your creative work, you can eliminate distractions and build momentum in your creative process. By following the steps outlined in this chapter, you can begin to establish habits that support your artistic vision and create a more productive and fulfilling creative life.

Maintaining Habits for Life:
How to Keep Up Your Progress Over Time

Congratulations! You've successfully built new habits that have improved your life in many ways. You have more energy, focus, and productivity. You're healthier, happier, and more connected to the people and activities you care about. But how do you make sure that your new habits stick for the long term? In this chapter, we'll explore some strategies for maintaining habits for life.

The first step in maintaining your habits is to acknowledge that this is a lifelong journey. Habits aren't something you can build and forget about. They require ongoing effort, attention, and commitment. However, the good news is that over time, habits become easier to maintain. Your brain has rewired itself to support your new habits, and they start to feel like second nature.

One important strategy for maintaining habits is to make them part of your identity. When you identify as a healthy eater, an early riser, or a regular exerciser, you're more likely to stick to those habits. This is because you see yourself as the type of person who does these things, and you don't want to let yourself down. Make your habits part of your personal story, and you'll find it easier to maintain them over time.

Another strategy is to track your progress. Regularly monitoring your habits helps you see how far you've come and motivates you to keep going. Use a habit tracker or journal to record your progress, and set milestones or rewards for yourself when you hit certain benchmarks. This helps keep you accountable and reminds you why you started building these habits in the first place.

It's also important to be flexible with your habits. Life is unpredictable, and sometimes you'll need to adjust your habits to fit your changing circumstances. Don't beat yourself up if you miss a workout or eat an unhealthy meal. Instead, take it as an opportunity to learn and adjust your habits accordingly. Being flexible and forgiving with yourself helps you stay motivated and makes it easier to maintain your habits over time.

Another key strategy is to find support and accountability. Habits are easier to maintain when you have a community of people who support and encourage you. Find a workout buddy, join a cooking class, or start a meditation group. Being around like-minded people who share your goals helps you stay motivated and inspired.

Finally, don't forget to enjoy the journey. Habits are a means to an end, but they're also an end in themselves. Building positive habits should bring joy, satisfaction, and a sense of purpose to your life. Don't get so focused on the destination that you forget to enjoy the ride. Celebrate your successes, learn from your failures, and savor the small moments of progress along the way.

In conclusion, building new habits is an ongoing process that requires commitment, flexibility, and self-compassion. By making your habits part of your identity, tracking your progress, being flexible, finding support, and enjoying the journey, you can maintain your habits for life. Remember that habits are a powerful tool for personal growth, and the effort you put into building them is well worth it. Keep up the good work, and enjoy the benefits of your positive habits for years to come!

....
END